Turning Back Time

The Ultimate Guide to Age Reversal After 50

by

Don Brown

Contents

Introduction

For those crossing the half-century mark, the quest to not only add years to life, but life to those years, has never been more achievable. This book unveils the art and science of reversing the clock, introducing you to the best methods and products at the forefront of age reversal. As we unfold the layers of understanding aging, nutrient-rich diets, exercise regimens tailored to mature bodies, and insightful mental health strategies, our mutual journey will provide you with the knowledge to rejuvenate your essence. It's about nurturing a youthful spirit and ensuring that your later years are lived to their fullest potential. Embrace the coming pages as your comprehensive blueprint to a revitalized and reinvigorated self, and let's embark on this transformative odyssey together. You will find the last two sections of Chapter 2, to be most useful in helping you to find not only the latest anti-aging products and techniques, but also how to keep up-to-date on the latest products, techniques and services.

Understanding the Aging Process

The journey through life brings with it changes and adaptations, and grappling with the aging process is something each one of us will confront. Understanding what aging genuinely entails is fundamental in transforming our later years into a period of growth rather than decline. The science behind aging is intricate and yet fascinating; it's not just about the years piling on but also about the biological and physiological shifts that occur over time. Every cell, every organ, and every system in our bodies encounters a gradual shift from growth to maturity to decline. This chapter delves into the biology of aging – the roles of genetics, the impact environmental factors have, and the complex interplay that determines how quickly or slowly we age.

It's essential to distinguish between the myths and realities that circulate about growing older. We confront an onslaught of stereotypes about aging, which range from the benign to the genuinely harmful. For instance, it's a common misconception that old age is synonymous with poor health or cognitive decline. However, new research suggests that with proper lifestyle adjustments and interventions, many aspects of the aging process can be slowed down or even reversed. Let's dispense with the fiction that aging is a downward spiral and instead focus on the myriad of opportunities for maintaining and even enhancing our vitality. We'll examine how adopting a proactive stance on aging can fundamentally alter our experience of life's later chapters.

As we delve into the realms of cellular senescence and telomere shortening, it's crucial to view these biological processes not as inescapable curses but as challenges that modern science is increasingly learning to mitigate. Today's advancements in age reversal are not just science fiction but a burgeoning field filled with promising methods and products. From innovative dietary strategies to lifestyle choices rooted in cutting-edge research, we're at the threshold of a new era where aging isn't something we passively accept but actively manage. By gaining a robust understanding of the aging process, we can lay the groundwork for the transformative techniques discussed in upcoming chapters, aimed at rejuvenating both body and mind.

The Science of Aging

As we delve deeper into the journey of aging, an understanding of its scientific intricacies becomes essential. Aging isn't merely a result of the passage of time; it's a biological process influenced by a symphony of molecular events. At the cellular level, aging can be described as the gradual accumulation of damage to cells, tissues, and organs, eventually leading to functional impairment. This damage accrues due to a variety of factors, ranging from genetic predispositions to environmental assaults. Key players in this process include telomeres, the protective caps on our chromosomes which shorten with each cell division, and oxidative stress, resulting from an imbalance between free radicals and antioxidants. Knowledge of these biological underpinnings arms us with a foundation upon which we can build strategies that may not just slow aging, but in some instances, possibly reverse its effects.

It's important to recognize that aging is a highly individualized process, governed by a complex interplay of factors such as genetics, lifestyle choices, and chronic stress exposure. Research has illuminated pathways such as the insulin/IGF-1 signaling pathway, which deeply influences longevity across various species. Moreover, the role of mitochondrial function cannot be overstated; these energy-producing organelles decline in efficiency with age, and their dysfunction is linked to a host of age-related conditions. By understanding these critical pathways, we can target them through precise lifestyle interventions, emerging pharmaceuticals, and even natural compounds that promote cellular rejuvenation and vitality.

Within this scientific framework, many have sought the proverbial "fountain of youth." The rise of senolytics, drugs that selectively clear away senescent cells that accumulate with age and contribute to chronic inflammation, offers a glimpse into the future of age reversal technologies. Factor in advancements in stem cell therapy, the potential of epigenetic reprogramming, and the exploration of the gut microbiome's influence on age-related diseases, and the horizon for reversing the aging process seems promising. While there are no guarantees, it's these scientific findings and innovative interventions that may allow individuals to enhance their healthspan, living healthier, more vibrant lives well past 50.

Common Myths and Realities of Growing Older

Much of what we think we know about aging is steeped in misconception rather than scientific reality. A ubiquitous myth is that sharp cognitive decline is an inevitable aspect of getting older. While it's true that certain cognitive functions can be affected with age, a multitude of studies have shown that the brain retains the remarkable ability to grow and change well into our later years—a concept known as neuroplasticity. This information is empowering because it means that engaging in cognitive exercises and adopting a brain-healthy lifestyle can significantly moderate the changes many fear as an unalterable consequence of aging.

Another prevalent fallacy is that the loss of muscle mass and strength—sarcopenia—is a predetermined outcome of aging. However, the reality is far from this defeatist view. Resistance training, protein-rich diets, and certain supplements can play pivotal roles in maintaining and even improving muscle strength as we age. By understanding the tools we possess, we can combat the complacency that often accompanies these aging myths and actively work towards optimal physical health. Remaining informed about cutting-edge products and methods helps older adults to challenge these misconceptions, promoting a proactive approach to longevity and age reversal.

Equally as important to dispel is the myth that emotional well-being declines with age. While it's undeniable that aging presents its own set of emotional challenges, such as dealing with loss or potential isolation, many people in their later years report higher levels of life satisfaction compared to their younger counterparts. The experiences and wisdom gained over a lifetime can contribute to a more resilient outlook. Hence, we understand that growing older doesn't necessarily mean growing disheartened. The aim, then, is not just to correct these myths but to embrace the strategies that lead to a rich, vibrant, and fulfilling third act of life.

Chapter 2: Nutrition for Longevity

As we move beyond our understanding of the aging process from Chapter 1, it's time to delve into one of the pivotal elements of age reversal: nutrition. The food we consume plays a critical role in not just maintaining, but enhancing our vitality as we age. It's about more than just eating well—it's about making strategic choices that can ignite the body's innate healing mechanisms and promote longevity.

Superfoods are not mere buzzwords; these power-packed sources of nutrition are essential for anyone looking to turn back the clock. The adage "you are what you eat" resonates profoundly when talking about age reversal. This chapter isn't about elusive or exotic ingredients but focuses on readily accessible foods that are rich in antioxidants, healthy fats, vitamins, and minerals. Incorporating these foods into your daily diet can help protect your cells from oxidative stress, reduce inflammation, and provide the raw materials needed for cell repair and regeneration.

Building an anti-aging diet plan isn't about restrictive eating; it's about finding balance and nourishing your body in a sustainable way. Tailoring your meal plan with an emphasis on plant-based foods, lean proteins, and complex carbohydrates can lead to improved energy levels and cognitive function. Don't worry; this isn't about revamping your culinary habits overnight. It's about making incremental changes that add up to a profound impact on your health and well-being over time.

While a solid diet is the foundation of age reversal, cutting-edge supplements and products can offer an additional boost. These products can range from advanced formulations that support metabolic health to novel compounds designed to enhance cellular repair. However, with the vast sea of supplements available, discernment is key. This chapter will navigate these waters, pointing you toward reputable sources that back their claims with solid research and where to find them without falling prey to the latest fads.

The journey toward a youthful existence doesn't end here. As integral as nutrition is, it represents one piece of a larger puzzle. The path to reclaiming and sustaining youthfulness also ventures into fitness routines, mental health strategies, and medical advancements—all of which will be discussed in subsequent chapters. For now, grasp the role nutrition plays in extending your health span and consider the power on your plate as the first line of defense against the toll of time.

Superfoods for Age Reversal

Turning back the hands of time isn't just a wishful thinking, it starts on your plate. The power of certain foods to support youthfulness and combat the aging process can't be overstated. Superfoods, packed with antioxidants, healthy fats, and vital nutrients become paramount as we surpass the age of 50. Let's navigate through some of these dietary heroes whose consumption may not only add years to your life but also life to your years.

Berries, such as blueberries, strawberries, and raspberries, are often celebrated for their high antioxidant content. These compounds are vital for combating oxidative stress, a key factor in aging and chronic disease formation. Introducing a variety of berries into your diet can help improve cognitive function and maintain healthy skin. Just imagine the countless ways you could incorporate them into your meals, from a refreshing morning smoothie to a mixed berry salad at lunch.

Another linchpin in your anti-aging arsenal should be leafy greens like spinach, kale, and swiss chard. They are rich in vitamins A, C, E, and K, as well as iron and calcium. These nutrients work in tandem to preserve bone health, maintain vision, and support cell regeneration. Often the heroes behind the scenes, these greens can easily find their place in your daily diet, from an omelet to a hearty dinner stir-fry.

Omega-3 fatty acids are key players too, which is why foods like salmon, walnuts, and flaxseeds can't be overlooked. Omega-3s support heart health, reduce inflammation, and play a crucial role in brain health. Incorporating them can mean choosing salmon for dinner instead of red meat and opting for a handful of walnuts as a snack rather than reaching for processed goodies.

Lastly, the importance of hydration and fiber is often underappreciated. Superfoods that are also high in water content and fiber, such as cucumbers and avocados, promote digestion and toxin elimination, which in turn can lead to better skin and energy levels. Avocados not only offer heart-healthy fats but also pack a fiber punch that keeps your digestive system running smoothly. By consciously choosing to include these foods in your diet, you're setting the stage for a body that feels and looks rejuvenated from the inside out.

Crafting Your Anti-Aging Diet Plan

As we continue to explore the pivotal role of nutrition in promoting longevity, it's vital to shift focus towards the practical application of these principles in your daily life. Crafting your anti-aging diet plan isn't just about selecting the right foods; it's weaving a tapestry of eating habits that nurture your body while warding off the effects of aging. Balance is key, and a well-structured diet plan should provide an abundance of vitamins, minerals, and antioxidants to bolster your natural defences and enhance cellular regeneration.

The foundation of such a diet is built upon whole, minimally processed foods. Think colorful fruits and vegetables, which are high in antioxidants that help neutralize free radicals – harmful byproducts of metabolism linked to the aging process. Leafy greens like spinach and kale, berries, and other vibrantly hued produce can become your new best friends. Quality protein sources are also crucial, particularly lean meats, fish rich in omega-3 fatty acids, and plant-based proteins like lentils and chickpeas. These nutrients are essential for maintaining muscle mass and promoting a healthy immune system as you age.

Incorporate healthy fats into your diet, focusing on those found in nuts, avocados, and olive oil. These fats are not just beneficial for your heart; they also aid in the absorption of fat-soluble vitamins crucial for skin health and cognitive function. While you're at it, be sure to stay hydrated. Adequate water intake supports every system in your body and helps maintain skin elasticity – a simple yet effective anti-aging measure. Aim for a balanced intake of complex carbohydrates as well, such as those found in whole grains, as they provide sustained energy and are rich in fiber, helping with digestive regularity and metabolic health.

While planning your diet, remember that portion control is just as important as food selection. With metabolism often slowing down as one ages, it becomes more necessary to match caloric intake with energy expenditure to avoid weight gain. Introduce variety to prevent nutritional deficiencies and to make your meals more enjoyable. Herbs and spices not only enliven your dishes but are also packed with anti-inflammatory compounds, which can further help in mitigating age-related conditions.

Lastly, it's wise to have an understanding of how your body's nutritional needs change over time, and adjust your diet accordingly. Consulting with a dietitian or utilizing online resources can provide tailored advice suited to your health status and lifestyle. Remember, it's not solely about longevity, but also about enhancing the quality of your life as you age. As you implement these dietary adjustments, you're setting a strong foundation for your body to thrive in its later years, ensuring that you can enjoy life to its fullest with vitality and vigor.

**The Latest Cutting-Edge Anti-aging Products &
Supplements and where to obtain them:**

1. Pure Kana: https://purekana.com/collections/

2. Organixx: https://shop.organixx.com/products/clean-sourced-collagens-20-servings

3. Verovital GH3: https://Realgh3.com

4. L'evateYou: https://levateyou.com

5. Boomerboost: https://boomerboost.com

6. Natural T boosters:

    "Best Testosterone Boosters | What's Legit And What Isn't!":

https://centertrt.org/Best-Testosterone-Boosters.html - https://www.testofuel.com/en-ca/ - https://umzu.com/products/testro-x

7. Reactivate: https://reactivateskin.com

8. High Impact Protein: https://www2.mypowerlife.com/os230601a_ap

9. High Impact Endurance: https://www2.mypowerlife.com/os210903a_ap

10. Age Reversal: https://Bioactivec60.com

11. Vision Health: https://visifreenow.com

12. Health Longevity:
https://paragonhealth.co/products/nmn500

13. Dermal Repair Complex:
https://lp.innerskinresearch.com/product-v02/index-v05-3287.html

14. "Home– PlantSynergy":
https://plantsynergybeauty.com

15. Muscle building and fat burning:
https://www.ultimateabs360.com

16. Resolitrol: https://resolitrol.com/product/resolitrol/

17. BioSkin Youth Complex:
https://www2.gundrymdbioskin.com/os220603a_ap?sessionid=9520513346&uid=aff_yt_bs_surveystart_220307&step=2

18. EIR Vitality Formula:
https://store.eirsupplements.com/products/quantum-all-natural-longevity

https://eirsupplements.com/breakthrough/

19. Springs Rejuvenation:

"Stem Cell Therapy | Peptides | IV Drips | Regenerative MedicineSprings Rejuvenation | Stem Cell & Regenerative Medicine Center":
https://springsrejuvenation.com

20. Qualia Senolytic: https://neurohacker.com/qualia-senolytic-asprey-details

21. Keranew: https://haircarereimagined.com/230313a/os/os.php

22. Pure NMN: https://donotage.org/product/pure-nmn/

23. Advanced Memory Formula: https://www.advancedbionutritionals.com/FB/Advanced-Memory/Nobel-Prize-Winning-Memory-Breakthroughs/SL-TPS.htm

24. Shilajit:

Blisque – Pure Himalayan Shilajit Resin Supplement | Authentic, Natural, and Organic | For Detox, Cleanse, Immune Support, Brain Booster and Energy | Contains Fulvic Acid and Trace Minerals: https://a.co/d/iTKaUj5

https://www.amazon.com/s?k=Shilajit&link_code=qs&sourceid=Mozilla-search&tag=mozilla-20

25. Armra Colostrum: https://tryarmra.com/
26. Bee Venom Face Serum: https://shorturl.at/uCOUY
27. Infinate Age Sea Moss: https://shorturl.at/iovHX

Above information is updated with clickable links at: AgeReversalPortal.com

It is important to keep **up-to-date** on the *latest* **anti-aging breakthroughs**. The following website portal has been created to help you to do so. Be sure to check the site periodically for the latest products, services and information:

http://www.agereversalportal.com

Chapter 3: Physical Activity and Its Role in Rejuvenation

Moving from the foundation of nutrition in the previous chapter, we turn our attention to the revitalizing power of physical activity. It's well-established that exercise is beneficial at any age, but after 50, it becomes critical for reversing signs of aging and promoting vigor. Yet, the question isn't whether to exercise, but how to tailor activities to maximize their rejuvenating effects. Engaging in regular physical activity not only helps maintain muscle mass and supports cardiovascular health, it can also enhance mental agility and elevate mood. But it's not just about hitting the gym or running marathons; the key is to find sustainable exercises that invigorate without overwhelming, building strength, and resilience while guarding against injury.

Imagine the possibilities when workouts are not merely a chore, but a source of renewal. Recent studies underscore that moderate, consistent exercise may trigger biological processes akin to a fountain of youth. When designed intelligently, exercise routines can maintain and even improve flexibility, which tends to diminish with age, and bolster balance to prevent falls—common concerns for those over 50. There's no need for high-impact moves that can stress the body; rather, a focus on activities such as brisk walking, swimming, or yoga can open the door to newfound vitality. Embracing a variety of exercises not only keeps the routine interesting but ensures a comprehensive approach to rejuvenation, engaging different muscle groups and promoting overall well-being.

Thus, physical activity stands as a pillar of age reversal, with its influence stretching beyond the confines of the gym. It imbues life with energy and zest, fortifying the body's defenses against the wear of time. For individuals over 50, this translates into an actionable plan that promises not just longevity, but a zestful and dynamic existence. Throughout the following sections, we dig deeper into specific exercise routines designed to foster youthfulness and explain how incorporating flexibility and balance training can further enhance the rejuvenation process. Armed with the right knowledge and strategies, the journey to a rejuvenated self is not just attainable—it's an exhilarating path forward.

Exercise Routines to Foster Youthfulness

Staying active is a cornerstone of a vibrant and youthful life, especially after 50. It's about more than just keeping the body in motion; it's about crafting exercise routines that are both sustainable and effective at maintaining vigor. Strength training, for instance, isn't merely about building muscle—it's also about preventing muscle loss, improving metabolism, and supporting bone density. By focusing on resistance exercises that target major muscle groups, individuals can tackle age-related muscle decline head-on. If hitting the gym isn't appealing, resistance bands and bodyweight exercises can also do wonders and can be executed within the comfort of one's home.

Cardiovascular fitness is equally essential in promoting a youthful essence. Activities like walking, swimming, or cycling are exceptional for heart health, endurance, and even mental clarity. For a holistic approach, it can be beneficial to alternate between different types of cardio throughout the week to engage various muscle groups and stave off monotony. What's crucial is finding a rhythmic exercise routine that not only challenges the body but also brings joy and can be eagerly anticipated—a dance class, perhaps, or a brisk early morning jog in the park.

Of course, one must never overlook the rejuvenating power of yoga and Pilates, which focus on core strength, flexibility, and breath control. These practices encourage a harmonious connection between body and mind, and they can be uniquely comforting as the body changes with age. Integrating these activities a few times a week can substantially enhance posture, reduce joint pain, and improve balance—a key aspect in preventing falls and maintaining independence. By combining strength, cardiovascular, and flexibility exercises, individuals over 50 can curate a comprehensive fitness routine that inherently celebrates and invigorates their youthful spirit.

Incorporating Flexibility and Balance Training

As we advance through the chapters of rejuvenation and self-care, a noteworthy dimension that oftentimes receives less limelight but is crucial for those over 50, is flexibility and balance training. The importance of these practices can't be overstated as they are critical for maintaining an active lifestyle, preventing falls, and participating in day-to-day activities with ease. Integrating flexibility exercises such as stretching or yoga can enhance your range of motion, decrease the risk of injury, and relieve muscle tension. Balance exercises like Tai Chi, standing on one leg, or using balance boards not only bolster stability but also contribute to cognitive improvements due to the concentration and coordination they require.

The incorporation of flexibility and balance routines into your daily regime will not only assist in sharpening reflexes but also in fostering a harmony of movement that can rejuvenate both body and spirit. Start small, with short sessions, and progressively build up. It's essential to listen to your body and adjust accordingly, especially if a particular movement causes discomfort. Bear in mind, consistency is key. A few minutes a day devoted to these exercises can lead to significant progress over time. Remember, you're not just training your muscles and joints, but also nurturing your nervous system and enhancing your overall spatial awareness.

Lastly, finding the right motivation and guidance is important. Consider enrolling in a class that focuses on flexibility and balance, as this can provide a structured environment and the support of a community with similar goals. Many local community centers and gyms offer specialized classes for those over 50. Or, for those who prefer the convenience of their own home, there's a plethora of online resources and video tutorials specifically catering to flexibility and balance training. No matter the path you choose, incorporating this training into your lifestyle is a proactive step towards age reversal and maintaining your zest for life.

Chapter 4: The Power of Mindfulness and Mental Health

Having explored the pivotal roles of nutrition and physical activity in fostering youthfulness, it's crucial to focus on the garden of our inner landscape — our mental health. The capacity for mindfulness, which can be described as maintaining a moment-by-moment awareness of our thoughts, feelings, bodily sensations, and the surrounding environment, could be a golden key in the age reversal quest. For individuals over 50, mindfulness is more than a practice — it's a daily reinforcement of mental vigor and emotional resilience. Clinical studies showcase that individuals who engage in regular mindfulness exercises exhibit significant reductions in stress, anxiety, and depressive symptoms, all of which can accelerate aging. Embracing mindfulness practices isn't just about stress reduction; it's about creating a foundation for a more vibrant and engaged life.

Mindfulness goes hand in hand with mental health, particularly as one navigates the later stages of life. Being mindful enables us not only to mitigate stressors but also to enhance our cognitive faculties. As we age, staying mentally sharp is as important as maintaining physical health; after all, a keen mind propels an active life. By implementing cognitive exercises into our routine, such as strategic games, memory challenges, and puzzles, we can fortify the neural pathways in our brains. Moreover, engaging in creative pursuits like painting, writing, or music can stimulate neuroplasticity, which helps in maintaining a youthful brain. Maintaining a sharp mind can make the difference between merely aging and aging gracefully.

As we progress on this journey of rejuvenation, mental health remains a cornerstone of our overall wellness. It's no surprise that an integrative approach combining mindfulness with other lifestyle modifications leads to the most significant enhancements in quality of life and longevity. Regularly practicing mindfulness not only enriches our present moments but also paves the way to a future of clarity, focus, and emotional depth. These mental health practices are not just methods to cope with aging but powerful tools to reverse its effects, helping us reap the full benefits of the wisdom that comes with greater life experience.

Stress Reduction for Enhancing Longevity

Maintaining mental health is just as crucial as physical health, especially as we navigate the complexities of aging. Elevated levels of stress have been linked to accelerated cellular aging, meaning that effective stress management isn't merely calming; it's a pathway to longevity. Mindfulness, the practice of staying present and engaged with our experiences without judgment, is a potent antidote to the relentless pace and pressures of modern life. As individuals cresting the age of fifty, embracing mindfulness can lead to profound changes in stress levels and, by extension, overall health. Focused breathing exercises, meditation, and even simple daily habits like mindful walking can become cornerstones in constructing a more serene, stress-resistant lifestyle.

Chronic stress poses a silent threat, often exacerbating age-related health issues such as hypertension, diabetes, and heart disease. However, developing a routine that includes mindfulness-based stress reduction techniques can fortify the body's resilience against these ailments. Techniques like progressive muscle relaxation or guided imagery not only provide immediate relief but also have cumulative benefits. They help recalibrate the body's response to stress by dampening the 'fight or flight' reaction, thereby reducing the secretion of stress hormones such as cortisol. By integrating these practices into daily life, you're not just mitigating the physiological wear and tear of stress; you're underpinning your mental fortitude and emotional well-being, contributing significantly to a rejuvenated, revitalized life experience.

Moreover, it's imperative to recognize that the mind-body connection plays a pivotal role in aging gracefully. Tapping into the tranquility that mindfulness cultivates can lead to many positive outcomes, including better sleep patterns, improved immune function, and enhanced cognitive performance. For those past mid-century, consistent mindfulness practice could translate to a diminished risk of age-related cognitive decline, stronger social connections, and a more vibrant, engaged existence. In essence, by managing stress through mindfulness, one can add not just years to life, but life to those years, and the journey to longevity becomes as rewarding as the destination.

Cognitive Exercises to Keep Your Mind Sharp

Engaging the mind consistently with cognitive exercises is a central tool for those seeking not only to maintain mental acuity but to foster cognitive rejuvenation. As we've explored various factors contributing to a youthful spirit, it becomes clear that an agile mind is as valuable as a healthy body. Mental puzzles such as Sudoku and crosswords are more than mere pastimes; they're neurobics for the brain that enhance problem-solving and pattern recognition skills. Likewise, learning new skills or languages can stimulate neurogenesis, the creation of new brain cells, a process once believed to be impossible after a certain age. Experimenting with different types of brainteasers, or dedicating time to a new hobby, such as playing a musical instrument or painting, can do wonders for keeping the mind sharp and adaptive.

However, we should not overlook the impact of social interaction on cognitive function. Engaging in regular, meaningful conversations is akin to a dance of the intellect, where memory, comprehension, and critical thinking are practiced seamlessly. Social activities, whether they're organized group discussions, book clubs, or simply frequent gatherings with friends, compel us to stay mentally alert and reinforce our cognitive networks. Engagement in such activities can also stave off feelings of loneliness and depression, which can exert deleterious effects on mental health, especially in later years. Therefore, prioritize setting aside time for socialization as part of your routine for mental rejuvenation.

Finally, technology offers an array of digital exercises designed to challenge the mind in novel ways. From apps that offer memory training to platforms that provide tailor-made cognitive workouts, the digital sphere is rich with resources that one can employ at their convenience. Embracing these technologies not only enhances cognitive resilience but also ensures familiarity with digital tools, an important aspect of staying current in an ever-evolving world. Remember, the goal is to build and maintain a robust cognitive reserve, safeguarding against age-related decline and promoting a mentally fulfilling life. Consistency is key, so integrate these exercises into daily life to reap the greatest benefits for your cognitive health.

Chapter 5: Revolutionary Age Reversal Treatments

As we delve into the world of age reversal, it's essential to highlight the groundbreaking treatments that have redefined what it means to age gracefully. The advancements in this field aren't just cosmetic quick fixes; they represent a shift towards a more profound understanding of cellular health and longevity. Among these innovations, certain therapies have emerged as frontrunners, pushing the boundaries of what was once considered science fiction. Cellular regeneration techniques, for instance, utilize the body's own mechanisms to repair and rejuvenate tissue at a molecular level, effectively turning back the clock on aging.

Another remarkable area of progress is in gene therapy, where cutting-edge research has unlocked the potential to alter our genetic code to slow, stop, or even reverse aging processes. This is not a matter of mere speculation; clinical trials and extensive studies are continuously being conducted to ensure the efficacy and safety of such treatments. Even in their early stages, these therapies have shown tantalizing promise, offering a peek into a future where age-related decline is no longer an inevitability. As we explore these treatments further, we consider not only their transformative capabilities but also their ethical implications, ensuring that the pursuit of youthfulness remains responsible and aligned with the greater good.

Moreover, scientists are tirelessly working to engineer biocompatible materials that can repair or replace aging organs and tissues. This synergy of biology and technology exemplifies the pinnacle of age reversal research, laying the groundwork for a new era in medical innovation. In the subsequent pages, we will investigate the mechanisms behind these treatments, assess their practicality, and guide you towards informed decisions about integrating them into your own life. While these advancements continue to evolve, they mark a thrilling chapter in the quest for longevity, offering hope and revitalization to those eager to embrace the full spectrum of their golden years.

Breakthroughs in Anti-Aging Medicine

In recent years, the field of anti-aging medicine has witnessed remarkable breakthroughs that offer hope for those seeking to decelerate the clock on aging. Clinicians and researchers have been tirelessly working on understanding the underlying mechanisms of aging, leading to the development of therapies targeting everything from genetic regulators to cellular repair systems. One of the most promising areas of advancement is in the realm of senolytics, drugs designed to selectively target and eliminate senescent cells—cells that have stopped dividing and contribute to aging and age-related diseases. By reducing the burden of these dysfunctional cells, senolytics have the potential to improve overall healthspan and possibly reverse aspects of aging.

Another exciting development involves the use of peptides and growth factors in anti-aging treatments. Specific peptides can stimulate skin repair, increase muscle mass, and enhance immune function. These compounds, often administered via topical creams or injectables, are rapidly becoming popular for their efficacy and targeted approach to reversing age-related decline. Growth factors, particularly those derived from stem cells, are also being explored for their profound regenerative abilities, helping your body to heal and renew itself more effectively—much like it did in your younger years.

In conjunction with lifestyle changes and personalized medical approaches, these scientific advances are forging a future where aging is tackled at its biological roots.

Treatments that were once the realms of science fiction are now entering clinical trials, bringing us closer to translating lab discoveries into real-world, accessible therapies. As you venture into the next chapters that scrutinize the effectiveness of various products and treatments, retain this optimism: the research community is continuously uncovering novel ways to mitigate the aging process, enhancing both longevity and quality of life as we know it.

Evaluating the Efficacy of Popular Age Reversal Products

With an abundant array of age reversal products gracing the market, discerning which treatments can truly deliver on their promises is crucial for those eager to revitalize their youth. These products, ranging from topical creams to dietary supplements, often flaunt impressive claims, but it's important to look beyond the hype. One must verify the scientific validity behind these claims through a critical evaluation of research studies, FDA approvals, and documented outcomes. Anecdotal successes, while inspiring, can't substitute for rigorous clinical trials. Ingredients such as retinoids, antioxidants, and peptides are often spotlighted for their restorative properties, but effectiveness can vary significantly from person to person.

In addition to scrutinizing active ingredients, the delivery mechanism also plays a crucial role in the product's potency. For example, some compounds may degrade if not properly stabilized, losing efficacy long before they penetrate the skin's outer layer. It is wise to invest in products from companies that invest in research and technology to enhance bioavailability and ensure the active ingredients remain potent from bottle to skin. Peer-reviewed studies often shed light on which products rise above the rest, providing empirical evidence that can guide our choices. Consulting with healthcare professionals can also help navigate these waters, ensuring that any regime aligns well with one's personal health profile and targets specific aging concerns with precision.

Moreover, what sets exceptional age reversal products apart is their ability to deliver consistent, long-term results. Beware of miraculous instant fixes that do not address the underlying aspects of skin aging. True age reversal is a gradual process that supports the skin's natural repair mechanisms over time. Always remember, the most telling sign of a product's efficacy lies in its sustained ability to enhance skin texture, reduce fine lines, and improve overall skin health. Pricing, too, can be misleading; a hefty price tag does not always equate to superior performance. Ultimately, informed consumers who combine patience with a keen eye for evidence-backed solutions will discover the treatments that genuinely turn back the clock, offering more than just temporary cosmetic fixes but real, enduring rejuvenation.

Chapter 6: Enhancing Your Appearance

The pursuit of maintaining and enhancing one's appearance is as timeless as the ages, and attaining a youthful glow while respecting the maturity of one's years can be both empowering and rejuvenating. In this chapter, we explore strategies that are not only tailored to cater to the unique needs of those over 50 but are also at the forefront of dermatological innovation and aesthetic enhancement. A radiant complexion and revitalized appearance often begin with diligent skin care. To effectively turn back the clock, one must adopt a skincare regimen that addresses the specific concerns that arise with age, such as dryness, fine lines, and loss of elasticity. The market brims with products boasting transformative ingredients like retinoids, peptides, and antioxidants. It's crucial to sift through these options and select high-quality serums and moisturizers that truly benefit mature skin, promoting rejuvenation at the cellular level. Additionally, regular exfoliation helps to remove dead skin cells, allowing for better absorption of these rejuvenating products, and skin becomes more receptive to treatments that can restore a healthy glow.

While topicals can have a profound impact, certain non-surgical cosmetic procedures have gained popularity due to their ability to deliver more pronounced results with minimal downtime. Treatments like microneedling, laser therapy, and injectable fillers can redefine one's appearance by enhancing skin texture, volume, and overall facial structure. For instance, microneedling stimulates collagen production, essential for maintaining skin's firmness and smoothness. Laser therapies can address pigmentation issues and promote skin tightening, whereas fillers can restore lost volume, providing a subtler and more natural enhancement compared to surgical alternatives. It's imperative, however, to consult with accredited professionals who specialize in aesthetic treatments for mature clients, ensuring that the chosen procedures align with the individual's health profile and aesthetic goals.

Last but certainly not least, we can't overlook the role that a well-coordinated wardrobe and an updated hairstyle play in complementing one's rejuvenated skin and refreshed features. Aligning your personal style with contemporary fashion, while also maintaining a sense of timelessness, can bolster confidence and project vitality. The key is to find the balance between trends and classic styles, ensuring that every article of clothing or accessory chosen plays a part in reflecting the best version of oneself. In summary, enhancing your appearance after 50 is a multifaceted journey – incorporating advanced skin care, selectively choosing cosmetic procedures, and expressing oneself through fashion and style – all weaving together to create a refreshed, vibrant exterior that mirrors the youthful spirit within.

Skin Care Strategies That Turn Back the Clock

As we venture deeper into our golden years, our skin's resilience and youthful glow can begin to diminish, but this doesn't mean we can't reclaim a visage that brims with vitality. It all starts with hydration – the cornerstone of supple, youthful skin. A rigorous regime of moisturizing with products high in hyaluronic acid and ceramides can work wonders in plumping the skin and reducing the appearance of fine lines. A little-known secret is to look for products that contain natural oils like rosehip and argan, as they're not only hydrating but also rich in antioxidants to help protect skin from environmental damage.

Exfoliation is another key player; gentle, regular exfoliation removes the barrier of dead skin cells that clog the skin and uncovers fresh new cells below. This allows the deeper penetration of moisturizers and rejuvenating serums, such as those containing retinoids or vitamin C. While the use of retinoids should be tailored to one's skin sensitivity, they're unrivaled in promoting skin renewal and collagen production, which can lead to firmer, more youthful skin over time. However, with great power comes great responsibility – one mustn't overlook the need for daily broad-spectrum sunscreen to protect vulnerable new skin.

Falling in step with the advances in skincare, consider incorporating cutting-edge products with growth factors, peptides, and stem cells that have emerged on the market. These ingredients can send signals to our cells to remind them of their once youthful function, effectively encouraging them to behave more youthfully – a true turning back of the clock. Consulting with a dermatologist for a personalized skincare plan is invaluable, as they can recommend tailor-made strategies that accommodate your unique skin type and concerns. With the right products and a personalized approach, your skin can reflect the vitality and spirit you feel inside, casting a luminous, rejuvenated image back at you each morning.

Non-Surgical Cosmetic Procedures After 50

As we continue to explore ways to enhance your appearance beyond the half-century mark, it's important to recognize the powerful role non-surgical cosmetic procedures can play. These treatments offer significant benefits without the need for invasive surgery, and they have become increasingly popular among men and women seeking to maintain a youthful appearance. Chemical peels, for instance, work wonders in rejuvenating skin by removing the outermost layers, revealing smoother, more radiant skin beneath. Similarly, microdermabrasion is a less intense procedure that exfoliates the skin, helping to reduce the appearance of age spots and fine lines. Both options can stimulate collagen production – a vital protein that tends to diminish with age.

Injectables, such as Botox and dermal fillers, deserve a special mention for their powerful anti-aging effects. Botox relaxes the muscles responsible for creating wrinkles, delivering a smoother forehead and eye area while fillers can restore lost volume and diminish the prominence of wrinkles. These treatments are highly customizable, allowing you to target your specific concerns with precision and subtlety. Remember, your goal isn't to look like a different person but to enhance the best version of yourself. It's crucial to seek out skilled practitioners who understand the art of tailoring these procedures to achieve natural-looking results that honor your individual beauty.

Laser therapies and intense pulsed light (IPL) treatments are another frontier in non-surgical cosmetic technology

that can have transformative effects on your skin's texture
and tone. These innovative light-based treatments can
address various concerns, including sun damage,
hyperpigmentation, and redness. They work by stimulating
the skin's natural healing process, promoting a more
youthful glow. No matter which option you explore,
remember that maintenance is key. Non-surgical
procedures typically require follow-up sessions to sustain
their age-defying benefits. So, it's not just about choosing
the right procedure but also committing to a long-term plan
that keeps your skin looking its absolute best – fresh,
vibrant, and full of life.

Chapter 7: Lifestyle Changes for Sustained Youthfulness

Embarking on a journey towards sustained youthfulness requires more than just temporary fixes or sporadic attempts at healthful living; it demands a holistic reconsideration of lifestyle. As we age, the need for quality sleep becomes paramount in our quest to remain vigorous and alert. Proper rest recharges the body's cellular repair systems, supports cognitive functions, and balances hormones that regulate metabolism and stress. By committing to a consistent sleep schedule and creating an environment conducive to uninterrupted rest, you establish a foundation not only for longevity but also for a healthier, more youthful feeling every day.

Yet sleep alone can't work miracles if we ignore the power of genuine connections and the roles they play in our lives. Social engagement has been scientifically linked to better cognitive function, lower rates of depression, and even increased longevity. It's about fostering relationships that provide support, laughter, and a sense of purpose. Integrate regular interactions into your routine, whether through volunteer work, clubs, or simply maintaining friendships. In doing so, you're not just passing the time; you're enriching your years with quality experiences that contribute to a youthful essence—even as the calendar pages turn.

Change is constant, but how we adapt to it plays a critical role in managing the aging process. Ingraining these elements into your lifestyle is not about superficial adjustments; it's about forging lasting habits that become second nature, infusing every day with activities and patterns that reinforce your vitality. When sleep and social ties are treated as pillars of health, akin to diet and exercise, rather than as optional extras, the tapestry of your life becomes one that not only looks vibrant but feels profoundly so from the inside out. Embracing these changes does not just add years to your life; it adds life to your years.

Sleep Optimization for Better Health

Entering into the realm of rejuvenating slumber, we recognize that as our bodies age, sleep becomes a critical cornerstone for maintaining youthfulness and vitality. For those over 50, mastering the art of restorative sleep is an investment with tremendous returns. Sleep optimization begins with establishing a routine — consistency is key. Aim to go to bed and wake up at the same time every day, even on weekends. This regularity fortifies your body's internal clock and can significantly improve the quality of your sleep. To further enhance your sleep environment, pay keen attention to factors such as room temperature, which should be slightly cool, and minimize exposure to blue light from screens before bedtime as it can interrupt your natural sleep-wake cycle. Incorporating relaxation techniques such as meditation or gentle stretching before bed can also promote deeper, more restful sleep.

Yet, quality slumber isn't solely about the environment or routines; it's also inextricably linked to what you consume. Be mindful of your diet and its timing; eating large meals or certain types of food too close to bedtime can disrupt your body's natural settling-down process. Caffeine and alcohol are notorious for impeding a good night's rest and should be enjoyed in moderation, especially later in the day. Replacing them with soothing beverages like herbal tea can be a comforting prelude to sleep. To support your journey to restful nights, explore the latest age reversal products specifically designed to enhance sleep, such as advanced sleep trackers that provide personalized data to fine-tune your sleeping patterns or supplements designed to support the body's natural circadian rhythms.

Remember, sleeping well is a form of self-respect and plays a pivotal role in age reversal by bolstering immune function, enhancing mood, and sharpening cognitive abilities. Embrace sleep as a healing balm; it's during these critical hours of rest that your body repairs cellular damage and clears out toxins, possibly slowing down the aging process. By prioritizing sleep and treating it as a vital component of your anti-aging regimen, you create a foundation of health, allowing you to greet each day with renewed energy and focus, ready to embrace the joys of life's extended prime.

Social Engagement and Its Impact on Aging

The importance of social engagement as you age cannot be overstated. Engaging with your community, maintaining friendships, and cultivating new relationships are not only fulfilling but also paramount in decelerating the aging process. Interpersonal connections provide emotional support, reduce stress, and have been linked to longer lifespans with improved quality of life. A robust social network can motivate you to stay active, eat healthily, and maintain a positive outlook on life. Consider joining groups or clubs that align with your personal interests. Not only do these social structures provide a sense of belonging, but the stimulation of social interaction can help preserve cognitive function, keeping your mind as agile as your body needs to be.

Engagement doesn't mean you have to constantly surround yourself with people. Quality over quantity holds true when it comes to your social contacts. Intimate gatherings, meaningful one-on-one interactions, and being part of a community that shares your values and hobbies boost self-esteem and contribute to a sense of purpose in everyday life. Moreover, these connections often act as a safety net that many over the age of 50 find comfort and security in. Creating a structured social schedule can weave these experiences naturally into your routine, ensuring you reap the benefits of companionship without feeling overwhelmed.

It's also worth exploring the latest technologies designed to enhance social engagement. Online platforms and social media can serve as bridges to overcome physical distance, allowing you to connect with family, friends, and like-minded individuals worldwide with ease. Participation in online forums or virtual events not only broadens your horizon but provides a continuous learning environment which is vital for maintaining cognitive health. Thus, whether through face-to-face interactions or digital means, increasing your social engagement is a critical lifestyle change with profound effects on arresting and reversing the aging process.

Conclusion

As we figuratively close the book on our journey through the ever-evolving landscape of age reversal, we stand at the threshold of an empowering truth: aging is not a fate etched in stone, but a process we can actively influence. The insights and methods discussed from nutrition to groundbreaking treatments are beacons that guide us towards prolonged vitality and wellness. Recognizing that our later years can be marked by rejuvenation rather than decline is both liberating and motivating. The task of integrating the best methods for age reversal into one's life requires commitment, but it's a commitment that bears the ultimate reward—a quality of life defined by health, vigor, and engagement.

What you've encountered here—the nutritional wisdom, the physical regimens, the mindful practices, and the innovative treatments—constitutes more than mere advice. These are the pillars upon which a renewed lease on life is built. It's vital to approach these methods with a spirit of openness and a penchant for experimentation to discover what resonates most deeply with your personal needs and goals. Technological advancements in the realms of medicine and wellness are rapid and ongoing, and staying informed about these developments can ensure you remain at the forefront of the age-reversal movement.

In the autumn of one's years, every moment is precious, and the choices we make today dictate the vibrancy of our tomorrows. As you steward your health and appearance with the tools provided, may you do so in the spirit of joy and discovery that has no expiration date. The best methods for age reversal, now in your hands, await your action. Seize them and step forward into a future where each new dawn is met with anticipation and zest for life's boundless possibilities.

Appendix A

If you're intrigued by the transformative journey that lies ahead, you're likely ready to delve into further study and application. With an informed resolve, you have the power to harness state-of-the-art methodologies and turn the clock back on aging. What follows is a meticulously compiled list of resources — books, websites, and articles that have been pivotal in shaping the landscape of age reversal.

Recommended Reading and Resources

The literature in the realm of age reversal is expansive, but the value lies in identifying works that are both scientifically sound and practical in their application. Here you'll find a selection that satisfies these criteria, carefully tailored to empower you with knowledge beyond what's been discussed. Let this curated collection guide your continued exploration into a lifestyle that favors vitality and longevity.

1. **The Longevity Paradox**: How to Die Young at a Ripe Old Age by Dr. Steven R Gundry MD.

Dr. Gundry's insights into the dietary choices that promote cellular rejuvenation are revealing and actionable.

2. **Lifespan**: Why We Age—and Why We Don't Have To by Dr. David A. Sinclair.

This book underscores the genetic and lifestyle factors involved in aging and ways to counteract them.

3. **The Telomere Effect**: A Revolutionary Approach to Living Younger, Healthier, Longer by Dr. Elizabeth Blackburn and Elissa Epel.

A deep dive into the science of telomeres, components of our chromosomes that play a key role in aging.

4. **Ageless**: The New Science of Getting Older Without Getting Old by Andrew Steele.

Discover the breakthrough technologies and ideas that are changing what aging means.

While the above publications offer a wealth of knowledge, staying updated on the latest developments is equally important. As such, consider bookmarking websites dedicated to the latest in anti-aging research and news.

- *Life Extension Magazine*

Features the newest health and anti-aging advancements and protocols.

- *The National Institute on Aging*

An authoritative source for the latest research and guidelines on aging.

- *Aging Cell*

A peer-reviewed journal focusing on the molecular mechanisms of aging.

Embarking on this journey is not a conclusion but an ongoing process of revitalization. These resources are tools in your arsenal, consistently replenishing your understanding and providing fresh insights into your age-reversal journey. Whether it's the intricacies of molecular biology or practical lifestyle strategies, the knowledge is now at your fingertips, ready to be utilized in favor of a rejuvenated existence.

Recommended Reading and Resources

As you journey through the transformative process of age reversal, expanding your knowledge base is not just helpful; it's essential. Among the resources you'll find indispensable are meticulously selected books that delve into the science of aging, nutrition plans that promote long-term health, and the latest breakthroughs in anti-aging medicine. Look for titles by leading experts in gerontology and nutrition, ensuring that you're receiving information that's not only enlightening but also actionable. Engaging with these materials will offer you a richer understanding of the principles laid out in previous chapters and assist you in customizing a routines that resonate with your unique needs.

In addition to traditional books, the internet offers a treasure trove of constantly updated content. Bookmark online portals and websites dedicated to cutting-edge anti-aging information. These platforms feature articles, reports on emerging research, and reviews of products that are revolutionizing the field of age reversal. Such online resources are excellent for staying informed about new supplements, treatments, and technologies as they hit the market. Participating in forums and discussion groups can also offer community support and advice from peers who are navigating similar challenges and successes in their quest for youthfulness.

Lastly, be sure to keep an eye on authoritative journals and publications from esteemed health organizations. These often provide rigorously vetted studies, giving you insights directly from the forefront of scientific exploration into aging. With the wealth of information at your fingertips, you can remain confident in your decisions, reassured by the backing of solid research. Remember, the quest for age reversal is not just about embracing the newest trends but about making informed choices that contribute to a vibrant and fulfilling life as you gracefully advance in years.

Glossary of Terms

As we navigate through the intricate world of age reversal, understanding key terms and concepts is essential. Below, you'll find a carefully curated glossary designed to demystify the specialized vocabulary that we've encountered in our journey. Whether you're exploring the latest superfoods, embarking on a new exercise regimen, or considering state-of-the-art treatments to rejuvenate your body and mind, this glossary will be your trusty companion.

A

- **Age Reversal**: Refers to practices, treatments, and lifestyle adjustments aimed at reducing, halting, or reversing the biological processes associated with aging.

- **Anti-Aging Diet**: A nutritional plan focusing on foods shown to contribute to longevity and prevent age-related deterioration.

B

- **Balance Training**: Exercises designed to improve stability and prevent falls by strengthening the muscles that keep you upright.

- **Biological Age**: An estimate of an individual's age based on various biomarkers, as opposed to the chronological age.

C

- **Cognitive Exercises**: Activities or games that stimulate thinking and memory to maintain or improve mental function.

E

- **Efficacy**: Effectiveness; often used in context to describe the success of a particular treatment or intervention.

- **Environmental Factors**: External conditions such as pollution, UV radiation, and chemicals that can impact aging.

- **Exercise Routines**: A set plan of physical activities designed to maintain or improve health and fitness.

F

- **Flexibility Training**: Stretching and exercises that improve the range of motion of muscles and joints.

M

- **Mindfulness**: A mental practice that involves focusing one's awareness on the present moment, while calmly acknowledging and accepting one's feelings, thoughts, and bodily sensations.

N

- **Nutraceuticals**: Products derived from food sources with extra health benefits in addition to the basic nutritional value found in foods.

P

- **Phytonutrients**: Chemical compounds produced by plants that have been found to provide health benefits.

R

- **Rejuvenation**: The act of restoring youthfulness or vitality.

S

- **Sleep Optimization**: Techniques or habits intended to improve the quality of sleep, thereby promoting better health and potentially slowing the aging process.

- **Stress Reduction**: The process of identifying stressors and taking steps to decrease their impact on one's life.

- **Superfoods**: Nutrient-rich foods considered to be especially beneficial for health and well-being.

- **Supplements**: Products taken orally that contain a dietary ingredient intended to supplement the diet. These can include vitamins, minerals, amino acids, and herbs.

T

- **Telemedicine**: The use of electronic communications and software to provide clinical services to patients without an in-person visit.

- **Topical Treatments**: Creams, serums, or ointments applied to the skin surface for therapeutic benefits or cosmetic improvement.

With this glossary, you're now equipped with a firmer grasp of the lexicon that will unlock insights into maintaining vitality and embracing cutting-edge age reversal techniques. Whether tweaking your diet, introducing new physical activity, or considering innovative medical treatments, this reference will ensure these concepts are readily at your fingertips.